USMLE STEP 2 CK
Epidemiology
& Bio-Stats
(plus Preventive Medicine & Ethics)

In Your Pocket

✓ Study guide for the USMLE STEP 2 CK exam.

✓ Prepare for your shelf examination.

✓ Be ready for your inpatient rotation.

Gregory J. Fernandez M.D.

First Edition, 2016
Author & Editor: Gregory J. Fernandez, M.D.
Publisher: M.D. Educational Services
Peer-reviewer: Dr. Sanita Belgrave
Book Design: Marie Meyer and Di Freeze

Copyediting: Editage Cactus Communications

ISBN-13: 978-1530194445

ISBN-10: 153019444X

This book is gratefully dedicated to my wife. Thank you for your support and always being there for me. Thank you for your kindness, your devotion, and your endless selflessness support. I love you... Thank you mother, father, step-mother, brothers, friends, and family for all your encouragement and endless love. Best of luck to all the medical dreamers, the road is long and I hope my book helps you through this journey. All the best...

Epidemiology
Table of Contents

Contents, continued

Epidemiology & Bio-Stats

Study designs

Cohort study

➤ Can be either a **retrospective cohort study** (looking back in time) or **prospective cohort study** (looking forward in time).

- Prospective studies are a more powerful study design compared to retrospective studies.

- Retrospective studies tend to have more bias, as information is lost.

- Cohort studies compare exposed groups from non-exposed groups and follows them prospectively or retrospectively for the development of the disease.

➤ A prospective Cohort study measures the relative risk (RR) of developing a disease based on exposure over time to reach an end-point, the disease.

➤ The study compares the presence of disease (cases) and the absence of disease (controls).

- Cohort study is the only way to directly determine incidence.

➤ **Relative risk** = a/a+b ÷ c/c+d.

- Determines if exposure will increase the relative risk of disease.

Disadvantages: cannot study rare diseases, expensive study design, and requires a large sample size.

Cohort Studies

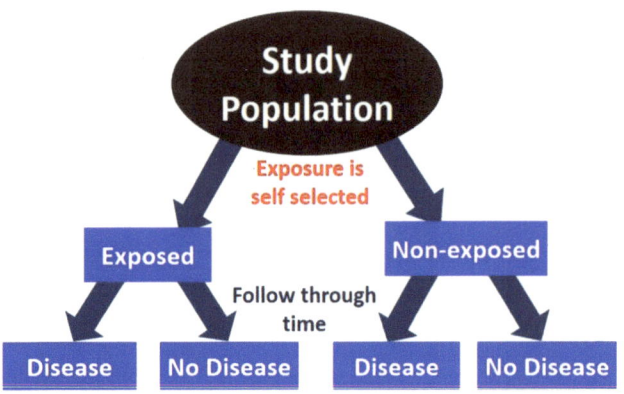

Source: howmed.net

Case-control study

➤ Only used for observational studies and retrospective studies to determine the odds ratio ($a \cdot d / c \cdot b$).

➤ Compares the presence of disease (cases) and absence of disease (controls) by studying previous exposure (retrospectively).

➤ Looks at the current outcome (disease) by retrospectively tracking previous exposure.

- Opposite of a prospective Cohort study: identifying exposure first → and then looking for disease in the future.

- Case-control: identifying disease first → and then monitoring previous exposure.

<u>**Advantages**</u>: can study rare diseases, inexpensive study design, fewer people needed, and can investigate an outbreak and quickly locate the source.

<u>**Disadvantages**</u>: cannot calculate disease prevalence, incidence, or directly measure RR.

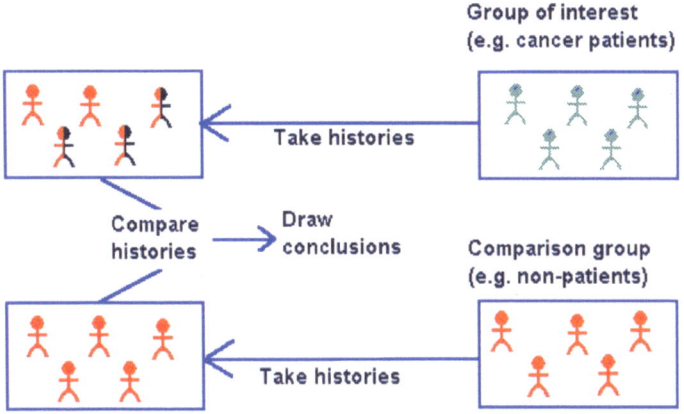

Source: library.downstate.edu

Longitudinal study

➤ A longitudinal study is an observational study in which data is gathered from the same subjects repeatedly over a period of time. Longitudinal studies can extend over years to decades. The same individuals are observed over a study period.

➤ Involves repeated observations of the same variables over long periods of time.

Clinical trial

➤ Clinical trial is a prospective study, similar in concept to a prospective cohort study.

➤ An experimental study that compares the benefits and side effects of two or more treatments.

➤ Basically studies the exposure of a medication and prospectively follows the patient over time to determine the outcome.

➤ Commonly uses numbers needed to treat.

➤ There are 4 phases involved in a clinical trial.

Crossover studies

➤ Is a type of longitudinal study where each subject acts as his or her own control.

➤ Can also be referred to as a crossover trial, in which the study participants receive different treatments in a random order.

➤ Crossover studies can limit confounding bias (a third variable that can alter the test results). Confounding is reduced because each crossover patient serves as his or her own control.

Cross-sectional study

➤ Is a "snap shot" study (one specific point in time) that is a cheap and easy study design.

  • Relatively quick and easy to conduct with no long periods of follow-up.

➤ Is an observational study where all factors (exposure, outcome, and confounders) are measured simultaneously.

➤ Can measure prevalence but cannot measure incidence.

➤ There is no timeframe in a cross-sectional study, as this is a snap shot of one specific point in time.

Cross-Sectional Research Study:

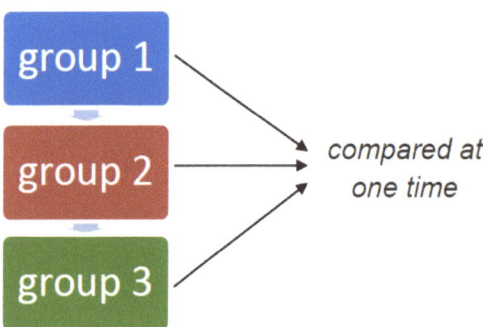

Source: study.com

Case report

➤ Looks at one case and does not compare with groups of subjects or controls. Commonly used for rare diseases.

➤ Case reports are considered to have the lowest level of validity and evidence.

Meta-analysis

➤ Has a high level of statistical power, validity, and evidence.

➤ Pooling data from several studies and combining them to achieve a greater statistical power.

➤ Usually, these studies will have a narrow confidence interval (CI), because an increased sample size corresponds to a tighter and more precise CI.

Blind studies

➤ A study design where the observers and/or subjects are unaware of which individuals or groups are subjected to the treatment or procedure variables.

➤ **Double-blind study:** neither the subjects nor the persons administering the experiment know the critical aspects of the experiment.

➤ **Single-blind study:** only the person administering the experiment knows of the critical aspects of the experiment.

➤ Single vs. double-blind study → single-blind study can lead to **procedure bias** or observational bias.

➤ Double-blind studies are better because this type of design prevents observational bias.

Latent period

➤ The time it takes a variable (the trigger) to have an effect on the disease.

➤ Is the time interval between the stimulus and response.

➤ Might need to study subjects for a longer period to determine outcome.

➤ Latent period is not a form of bias.

Effect modification

➤ When the effect of the exposure of interest on an outcome is modified by another variable.

➤ Is a <u>natural</u> phenomenon that should be described in the discussion section.

➤ Usually cannot eliminate effect modification and is <u>not</u> a form of bias, but can alter the results.

Randomization

➤ The goal is to create groups with a <u>similar</u> distribution of known and unknown variables; the only difference is the exposure variable in the study.

➤ Randomization helps decrease confounders in the study.

Bias types

Common types of bias

Measuring bias, recall bias, reporting bias, observer bias, selection bias, sample bias, late-look bias, lead-time bias, Pygmalion effect, Berkson's bias, Hawthorne effect, and confounding bias.

Measuring bias

➤ Can be caused by not using the same technique to measure, using a bad technique, mechanical error, or not recalling accurate information.

➤ Information is gathered in a way that alters or distorts the information.

➤ Random error is a non-systematic measurement error that is beyond our control.

Note: control groups or placebo groups help prevent measurement bias.

Recall bias

➤ Altered recollection of past events that create bias.

➤ Altered recall is more common in retrospective studies.

➤ Common in surveys.

Note: prevent recall bias by confirming information from others.

Reporting bias

➤ Involves a skew in the availability of data by selective revealing or suppression of information by the subject.

➤ A tendency to under-report unexpected or undesirable experimental results.

Note: prevent reporting bias by double blind study design.

Observational bias

➤ A type of bias where the investigator's evaluation is impacted by knowledge of the exposure status. Personal judgement may alter how the experiment is carried out or how the results are recorded.

Note: a double blind study design can decrease observational bias.

Selection bias

➤ Non-random assignment of individuals to the study group.

➤ If study design involves volunteers in the study this often leads to selection bias, as subjects volunteer commonly because of personal interests.

Note: randomization can be helpful to decrease selection bias.

Sampling bias

➤ Subjects are not representative of study design, which means the results are not generalizable.

Example: people willing to participate in studies because they have a family history.

- The individuals or groups in the study are selected in a way that randomization is not achieved.

Note: randomization can be helpful to decrease sample bias.

Late-look bias

➤ Information gathered at an inappropriate point in the timetable.

➤ When patients with severe disease do not get studied because of death.

Lead-time bias

➤ Detection of disease earlier; therefore, it appears that subjects are living longer.

- Bias is caused by improved screening technics.

➤ Gives false estimates of survival rates.

Pygmalion

➤ Describes the effects of researcher's beliefs on the outcome of the study, which can affects the overall outcome.

Note: double-blind study helps prevent this type of bias.

Berkson's bias

➤ Selection bias by evaluating data from hospitalized patients and comparing them to non-hospitalized patients.

Hawthorne

➤ Subjects behavior is altered or modified because they know they are being studied.

Confounding bias

➤ A third variable that can alter the test results (at least part of the relationship can be explained by another variable).

➤ A good way to prevent confounders is to create a good study design and use **stratified analysis**.

Note: ways to decrease confounding bias include randomization (matching controls by age and race, and selecting controls from the same neighborhood).

Biostatistics

Intention-to-treat

➤ The principle of intention-to-treat is the study is randomized.

➤ The approach is to provide unbiased comparisons among the treatment groups.

➤ In other words, everyone who is randomized in the trial is considered to be part of the trial regardless if they complete the trial.

Number needed to treat (NNT)

Number needed to treat (NNT) represents the number of patients over a given time period that one would need to be treated to prevent one additional bad outcome.

NNT = 1/absolute risk reduction (ARR).

➤ ARR is the difference in probability of disease among the exposed population (experimental/treatment group) and an unexposed population (control group).

➤ ARR = % - % = (control event rate) – (experimental event rate).

Example: if the (control event rate) is 20% and the (experimental event rate) is 25%.

• ARR = 20% - 25% = (0.20 – 0.25) = 0.05.

- NNT = 1/ARR = 1/0.05 = 20.
- NNT is equal to 20 → meaning you need to treat about 20 individuals to cure one person.

➤ Interventions that are more effective have a lower NNT number.

Example:

- If NNT= 1 → than everyone is cured by the intervention [perfect drug].
- If NNT = 10 → than 10 people need to take the drug to cure just one person [lower cure drug rate].

Note: ARR is the inverse of NNT.

Numbers needed to harm (NNH) = 1/attributable risk.

- NNH is a measure of how many patients on average need to be exposed to a risk factor over a time period to cause harm in an average of one patient who would not otherwise have been harmed.
- To determine **attributable risk** subtract incidence without exposure from incidence with exposure.
- NNH is the inverse of attributable risk.
- The lower the number need to harm, for example (3 verses 10), here 3 being the lower of the two numbers would mean this is a worse intervention than 10. Where 10 being the higher number, would mean you have to expose 10 individuals to develop one individual with an adverse outcome.
- This means that if 10 individuals are exposed to the risk factor, 1 will develop the disease that would not have otherwise.

Sensitivity

➤ This represents the patients who have tested positive for the disease or the probability of a subjects testing positive, in patients whom truly having the disease.

- In other words, is the probability of detecting the disease (true positives).

➤ Sensitivity = a/(a+c) or true positive (TP)/(TP + false negative [FN]).

➤ "SnOut" used to rule out disease (when the sensitivity test is negative) and identify sick people correctly (when the sensitivity test is positive).

➤ A high sensitivity test has few false negatives and is effective at ruling conditions "out" (SnOut).

➤ When a screening test has a sensitivity of 90% out of a 100 cases with the disease, the screening test detected approximately 90% of the patients who are TP and 10% who are FN (meaning they do have the disease, but it was not detected by the screening test). Basically, the screening test failed to detect 10% of the patients with the disease that should have been detected.

➤ Increase sensitivity = decrease false negatives = increase negative predicted value.

➤ High sensitivity equals high negative predictive value.

➤ Sensitivity is independent of the prevalence of the disease in question.

Note: used for a <u>screening</u> test (the higher the sensitivity, the better the screening test).

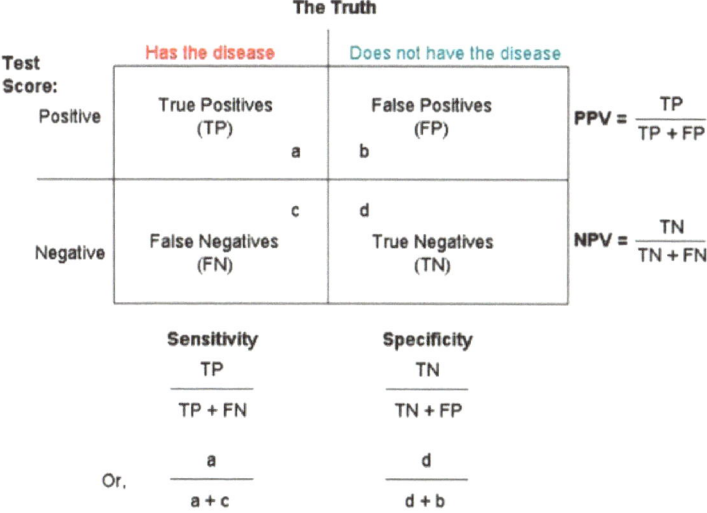

Source: www.med.uottawa.ca

Specificity

➤ d/(b+d) <u>or</u> true negative [TN]/(TN + false positive [FP]).

➤ Specificity represents the population that tests negative for the disease or the probability of testing negative in patients who do not have the disease (healthy patients).

  • In other words, specificity relates to the test's ability to correctly detect patients without a condition.

➤ While a highly sensitive test will say, 'we have a problem', a highly specific test can reliably say, 'its not the problem'. Therefore, specificity its very good at excluding.

➤ A high probability that a patient without a disease will have a negative test result, means the test is more specific.

➤ "SpIn" used to rule in disease (if positive test results) or healthy people correctly identified as healthy (if negative test results).

➤ A high specificity test has few false positives and is effective in ruling conditions "in" (SpIn).

  • A positive result in a test with high specificity is useful for ruling in disease.

➤ Increase specificity = decrease sensitivity.

➤ Increase sensitivity = decrease specificity.

➤ A test with a high specificity has a low type 1 error rate.

Note:

✓ Used for <u>confirmatory</u> test that is not affected by prevalence.

✓ A diagnostic test with perfect **validity** would have a sensitivity and specificity equal to 1.

✓ As specificity increases, the positive predictive value (PPV) increases, and the number of FPs decreases. You can determine what happened to false positives by looking at the equation.

✓ Specificity is inversely proportional to false positives.

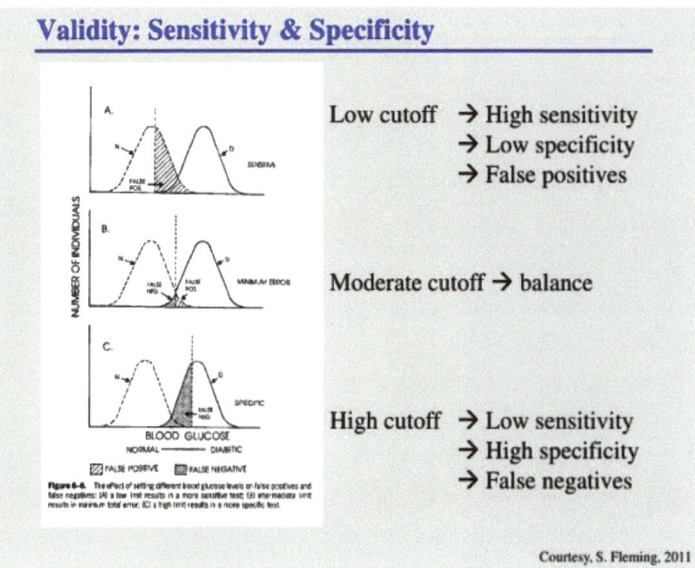

Source: www.slideshare.net

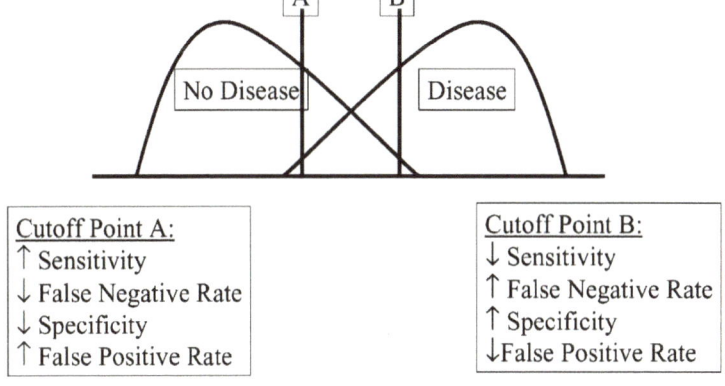

Source: jbjs.org

Bell-shaped curve representing sensitivity and specificity

➤ TN rate: represents specificity.

➤ TP rate: represents sensitivity.

➤ The furthest point to the <u>right</u> of the healthy curve represents 100% specificity.

➤ The furthest point to the <u>left</u> of the disease curve represents 100% sensitivity.

➤ If you move the vertical line (cutoff) to the <u>left,</u> specificity decreases and sensitivity increases.

  • Increased sensitivity would increase the number of TPs and decrease the number of FNs.

  • Increased sensitivity would decrease type II error and increase NPV.

➤ If you move the vertical line (cutoff) to the <u>right,</u> specificity increases and sensitivity decreases.

➤ Increased specificity would increase the number of TNs and decrease the number of FPs.

➤ Increased specificity would decrease type I error and increase PPV.

➤ If you move the vertical line (cutoff) to the left, the number of FPs increase.

➤ If you move the vertical line (cutoff) to the right, the number of FNs increase.

➤ Here again:

  • High sensitivity= low false negatives.

  • Low sensitivity = high false negatives.

  • High specificity = low false positives.

  • Low specificity = high false positives.

Note:

✓ True positive = correctly identified.

✓ False positive = incorrectly identified.

✓ True negative = correctly rejected.

✓ False negative = incorrectly rejected.

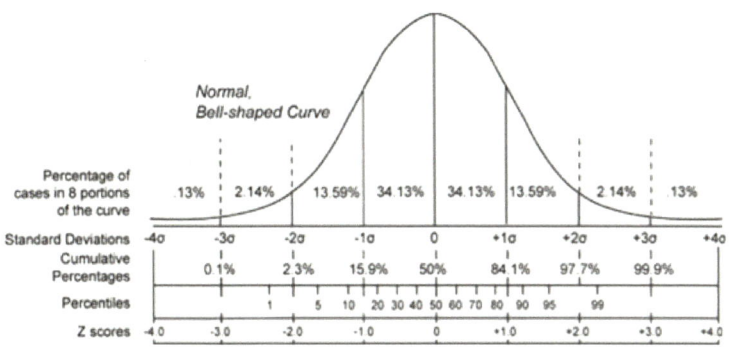

Source: ipscience-help.thomsonreuters.com

Positive predictive value (PPV)

➤ PPV = a/(a+b) or TP/(TP + FP) or (true positive) / (true positive + false positives).

➤ Represents the probability of having a condition given a positive test result.

➤ The more specific a test → than the higher the PPV.

➤ The less specific a test → than the lower the PPV.

Note: the higher the prevalence → the higher the PPV for that disease.

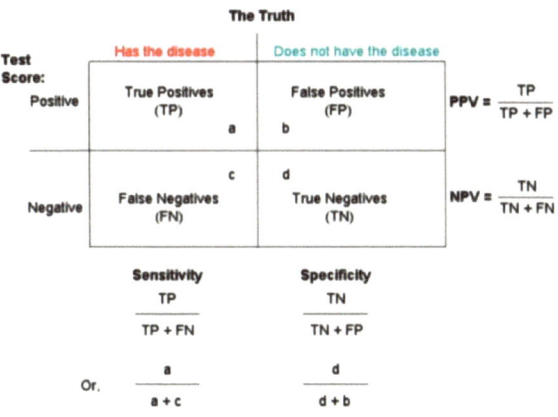

Source: www.slideshare.net

Negative predictive value (NPV)

➤ NPV = d/(c+d) or TN/(TN + FN) or (true negative) / (true negative + false negatives).

➤ Represents the probability of not having the disease given a negative test result.

➤ The more sensitive a test à than the higher the NPV.

➤ The less sensitive a test à than the lower the NPV.

Note:

✓ The lower the disease prevalence the the higher the NPV for the disease.

✓ NPV and PPV are essentially opposite regarding disease prevalence.

✓ Prevalence does not alter sensitivity or specificity.

Odds ratio

➤ (ad)/(bc) or (TP × TN)/(FP × FN).

➤ Odds of exposed in those with disease ÷ odds of exposed in those without disease.

  • In the numerator are the diseased and in the denominator are the non-diseased.

➤ Calculates the odds of how much more likely a person with a disease has been exposed to a risk factor than someone without the disease.

➤ Can use odds ratio to estimate relative risk for rare diseases.

➤ Odds ratio interpretation:

  • Odds ratio >1 than exposure is associated with a higher odds of disease.

  • Odds ratio equal to 1 than there is <u>no</u> association between the exposure and outcome.

  • Odds ratio <1 than exposure is associated with a lower odds of disease.

  • The larger the odds ratio the more impressive the study becomes.

> Used for **case-control studies** (case = with exposure; controls = without exposure).

  • Case-control studies are at greater risk of bias than Cohort studies.

Note: basically, studying a disease and retrospectively analyzing if exposure is what caused the outcome.

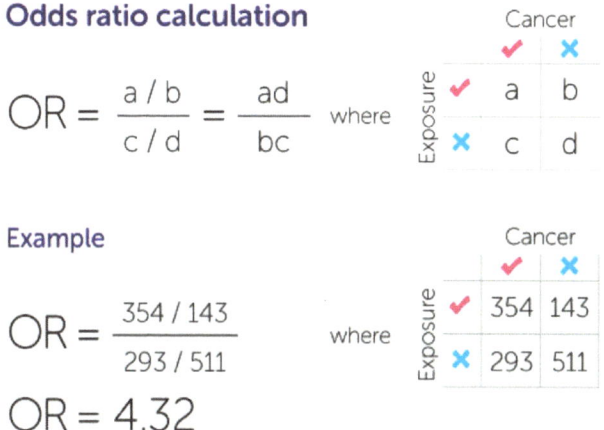

Odds ratio calculation

$$OR = \frac{a/b}{c/d} = \frac{ad}{bc}$$ where

Exposure	Cancer ✔	Cancer ✘
✔	a	b
✘	c	d

Example

$$OR = \frac{354/143}{293/511}$$ where

Exposure	Cancer ✔	Cancer ✘
✔	354	143
✘	293	511

$$OR = 4.32$$

Source: floroven.preschoolfirst.mob

Relative risk (RR)

> (a/(a+b)) ÷ (c/(c+d)) or (TP/(TP + FP))/(TN/(TN + FN)).

> Relative risk expresses how much more likely an exposed person is to get a disease compared with an unexposed person over a period of time.

> Relative risk > 1 means there is an increased risk of outcome.

> Relative risk equal to 1 means there is no risk of outcome.

> Relative risk < 1 means there is a decreased risk of outcome.

> The larger the relative risk the more impressive the study becomes.

> Calculating relative risk reduction (RRR) = [1-RR] x 100.

  Example 1: what is the RRR if the relative risk is = 1.45.

  • RRR = [1-1.45] x 100 = 45% *increased* risk of disease with exposure.

Example 2: what is the RRR if the relative risk is = 0.70.

- RRR = [1-0.70] x 100 = 30% *decreased* risk of disease with exposure.

➤ Used in **Cohort studies** (prospective study).

Note: basically, RR is the probability of the <u>exposed</u> group and the <u>unexposed</u> group to acquire the disease from the exposure of interest. The concept is to propectively monitor the exposure and determine if the disease develops.

*Relative risk is basically the probability:

- For example: what is the probability if out of 10 people, 6 of them have a heart attack. The probability is 6/10 = 0.60 or 60%.

- In the numerator is the exposed group and in the denominator is the total number of subjects.

- Probability will never be higher than 1.0 or 100%.

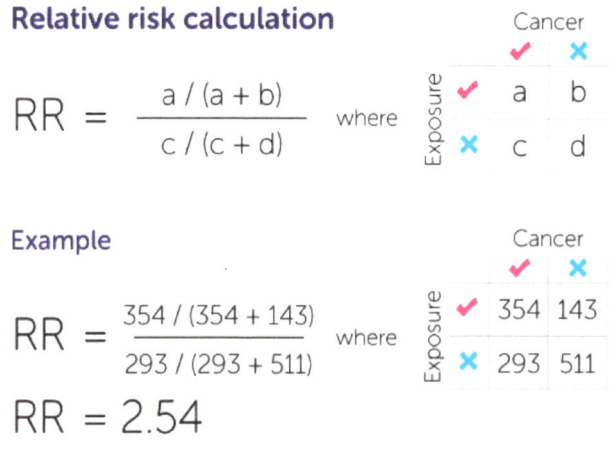

Relative risk calculation

$$RR = \frac{a / (a + b)}{c / (c + d)} \quad \text{where}$$

	Cancer ✔	Cancer ✖
Exposure ✔	a	b
Exposure ✖	c	d

Example

$$RR = \frac{354 / (354 + 143)}{293 / (293 + 511)} \quad \text{where}$$

	Cancer ✔	Cancer ✖
Exposure ✔	354	143
Exposure ✖	293	511

$$RR = 2.54$$

Source: www.cancerresearchuk.org

Attributable risk

➤ Attributable risk is the <u>difference</u> in the rate of a condition between the exposed and non-exposed groups.

➤ For instance, if the exposed incidence is equal to 50% and the unexposed incidence is equal to 25%, then the attributable risk is equal to 0.50 (exposed) – 0.25 (non-exposed) = 0.25 or 25%.

➤ **Attributable risk percentage** = attributable risk/exposed population. For example, in the above calculation, the attributable risk was calculated as 0.25 or 25%. Now, you divide the "attributable risk" by the percentage of the "exposed group," which was 0.50 or 50%. Then, we calculate the attributable risk percentage to be 0.25 (attributable risk)/0.50 (exposed group) = 0.50 or 50%.

➤ **Number needed to harm** = 1/attributable risk.

Prevalence

➤ Is the total number of new cases (incidence) and old cases at a given time, divided by the total population.

   • Another words, total cases in the population at a given time ÷ by total population.

   • Prevalence is usually expressed as a percentage, fraction, or by number of people.

➤ Chronic disease where treatment increases the survival rate would also increase the prevalence.

➤ As diagnostic testing becomes more specific, → the prevalence also increases.

➤ The higher the disease prevalence,→ the higher the PPV.

➤ Prevalence does not effect specificity or sensitivity.

➤ Cross-sectional studies and Cohort studies are a good way to determine prevalence.

➤ Types of prevalence:

   • Point prevalence is the proportion of a population with disease at a specific point in time.

   • Period prevalence is the proportion of a population with disease at a specific period in time.

• Lifetime prevalence is the proportion of a population that will have disease at some point in their life.

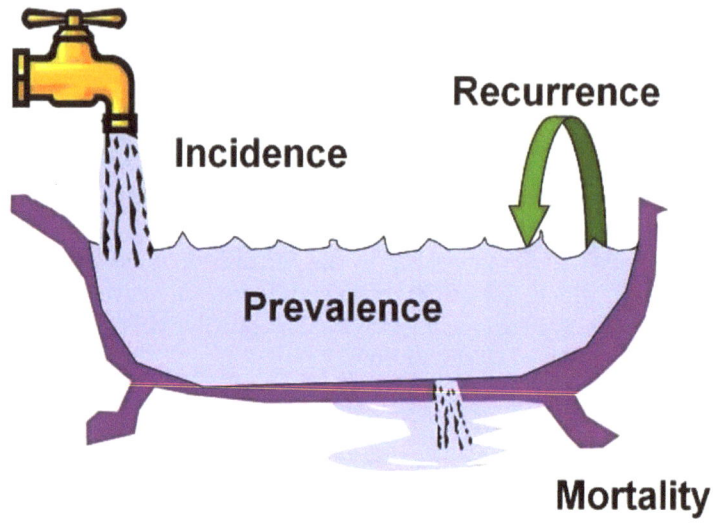

Source: www.pinterest.com

Incidence

➣ Is equal to new cases in the population over a given time period ÷ total population at risk during that time period.

➣ If the population is already diagnosed with a disease, this would not be included in the incidence; the incidence is the number of new cases, not cases that have already been considered.

➣ Primary prevention (vaccination, diet, and exercise) can decrease both the incidence and prevalence.

➣ Improved diagnostic testing can increase both the incidence and prevalence of a disease.

➣ Measures only new cases and would not be affected by prolonged survival secondary to treatment.

➣ Incidence can be measured by Cohort Study.

Note:

✓ Prevalence > incidence (for chronic disease).

✓ Prevalence = incidence (for acute disease).

Precision

➤ Is the consistency of the test: precision, reproducibility, or reliability ("PRR").

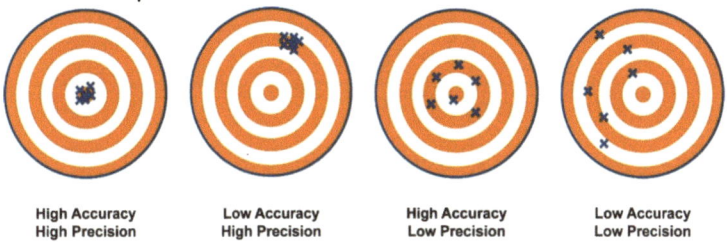

| High Accuracy | Low Accuracy | High Accuracy | Low Accuracy |
| High Precision | High Precision | Low Precision | Low Precision |

Source: http://climatica.org.uk/climate-science-information/uncertainty

Accuracy

➤ Is the trueness of the test: accuracy, trueness, and validity. ("ATV").

➤ A measurement system is considered valid if it has both accurate and precise.

Statistical distribution

➤ **Mean** = average number.

➤ **Mode** = most common number.

➤ **Median** (middle value) = the number in the middle of the variables.

➤ **Range** = the difference between the highest number and lowest number.

> **Example 1**: find the mean, mode, median, and range of these numbers: 2, 4, 6, 2, 8.
>
> • Mean is equal to the average of all numbers --> 2 + 4 + 6 +2 + 8 ÷ 5 = 4.4

- Mode is equal to the most common number --> the number 2 is present twice in the example.

- Median is equal to the number in the middle, when all numbers are arranged chronologically --> 2, 2, 4, 6, 8 than 4 is the median.

Example 2: if number set 17, 18, 20, 26, 27, 29, then the median would be in between 20 and 26, or 23.

- Range is the difference between highest and lowest numbers → 2, 7, 3, 5, 4, 8. Range 2-8 = 6.

Normal bell shape

In a normal standard bell shape curve: mean = median.

➤ 1st standard deviation = 68%.

➤ 2nd standard deviation = 95% (represents a Z-score of 1.96).

➤ 3rd standard deviation = 99.7% (represents a Z-score of 2.58).

➤ The total number under the curve is = 1 or 100%.

A normal standard bell curve needs to have equal division of the percentages to create a mirror image on both sides of the bell curve:

➤ -1 0 +1 (first standard deviation) → 34% fall on either side of zero.

- Total 68% with addition of 34% plus 34% (on either side).

➤ -2 -1 0 +1 +2 (second standard deviation) → 13% fall between -1 and -2 and another 13% fall between +1 and +2.

- Total 95% with addition of first and second deviation.

➤ -3 -2 -1 0 +1 +2 +3 (third standard deviation) → 2.14% fall between -2 and -3 and another 2.14% fall between +2 and +3.

- Total 99.7% with the addition of first, second, and third deviation.

Note: the **Z-score** tells you how many standard deviations a value is from the mean.

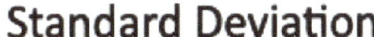

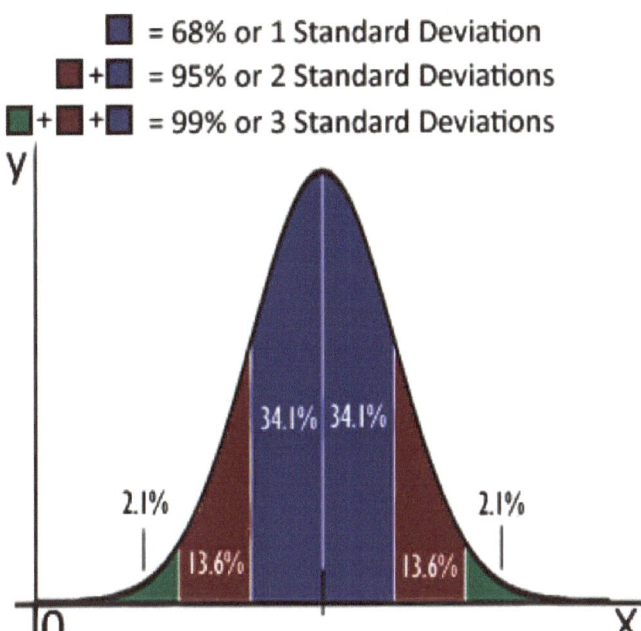

Source: www.valuewalk.com

Positive skew

➢ Mean > median > mode. Notice they are in alphabetical order.

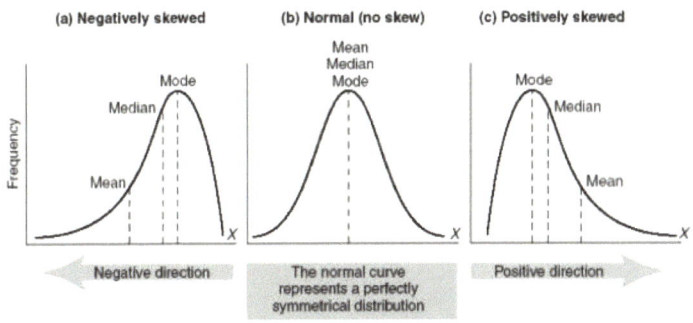

Source: www.thinglink.com

Negative skew

➤ Mean < median < mode. Notice they are in reverse alphabetical order.

Bimodal

➤ Is simply a 2-humped bell-shaped curve.

Null hypothesis (H0)

➤ States there is no difference or association between the disease and the risk factors in the population.

Alternative (H1)

➤ States there is some difference or association between the disease and the risk factors in the population.

Type 1 error (α)

➤ To accept there is a difference when none exists.

  • Another words, you accept the test results as true, when in fact they are false.

  • Or, accepting the experimental hypothesis and rejecting the null hypothesis (H0), when in fact the null hypothesis true.

➤ Type 1 errors are false positives (the test is positive but are really a negative event).

➤ If $p < 0.05$ there is less than a 5.0% chance of a false positive.

➤ The higher the specificity the lower the false positive rate and the lower the type I error.

➤ The lower the specificity the higher the false positive rate and the higher the type I error.

Note: p-value is the probability of making a type I error.

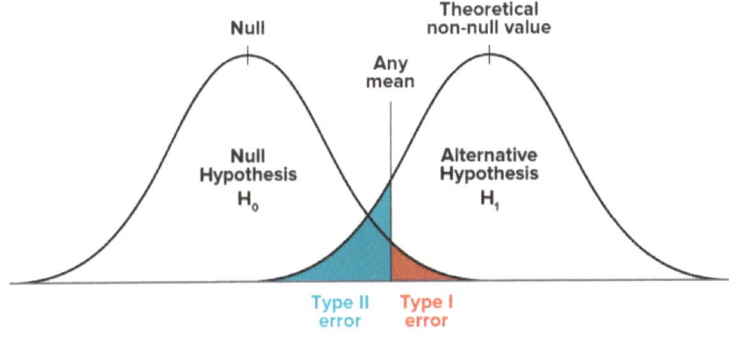

Source: grasshopper.com

Type II error (β)

➤ To accept that there is not an effect or difference when one exists.

➤ Accepting the null hypothesis, when in fact it is false.

  • Rejecting the experimental hypothesis, when in fact it is true.

➤ Type II error are the false negatives (testing negative but are really a positive event).

➤ The higher the sensitivity the lower the false negatives and the lower the type II error.

➤ The lower the sensitivity the higher the false negatives and the higher the type II error.

Power (1-β)

➤ Power is the probability of rejecting the null hypothesis when it is in fact false.

➤ Increase power with increased sample size and precision.

➤ Increasing power or sample size will decrease type II error.

➤ n = sample size.

➤ Sigma = standard deviation:

  • 1$^{\underline{st}}$ standard deviation = 68%. Meaning 68% of population lies within "one sigma".

- 2nd standard deviation = 95% (represents a z-score of 1.96). Meaning 95% of population lie within "two sigma".
- 3rd standard deviation = 99.7% (represents a z-score of 2.58). Meaning 99.7% of population lie within "three sigma".

➤ Standard error of the mean (SEM) = standard deviation/$\sqrt{}$ n (sample size).

- As the sample size increases SEM decreases.

➤ Confidence interval (CI): is a type of interval estimation of the population parameters. It determines the confidence that the true RR or odds ratio of repeated measures would be expected to fall within the interval.

- For example, if 95% CI for a RR is 1.5–2.5, there is a 95% chance that the actual RR will fall between 1.5 and 2.5.
- If confidence interval included 1.0 (example 0.8-1.5) than it is not significant, as 1.0 means there is no association.

➤ If RR or odds ratio is equal to 1.0, there is no association between the exposure and outcome.

➤ P-value is the probability of making a type I error.

➤ 95% CI corresponds to p-value = 0.05 or z-score of 1.96.

➤ P-value basically represents the probability of an H0 occurrence.

- For instance, if P = 0.01, there is only a 1% chance that the H0 is true.

➤ If p < 0.05 (considered statistically significant), there is a <5% chance that the H0 is true, and can reject the H0 and accept the alternative hypothesis under these circumstances.

- If p < 0.04, there is a <4% chance that in fact the H0 is true.

➤ If p > 0.05, the H0 can be accepted, and the findings are not statistically significant.

Note: the tighter the CI, the more power and confidence and the larger the population size. Confidence width is <u>inversely</u> proportional to sample size (as population size increases, the CI becomes tighter and more precise).

T-test (student's *t*-test)

➤ Measures the difference between the means of two independent groups.

➤ Is one of the most commonly used techniques for testing a hypothesis by comparing the difference between sample means.

➤ To conduct this test, you need to calculate the means or know the means of the two independent groups.

➤ If P < 0.05, reject the H0.

Paired *t*-test

➤ Is similar to the student's t-test, but measures and compares dependent means (not independent means). For example, the mean BMI of the same person before and after treatment.

Analysis of variance (ANOVA)

➤ ANOVA provides a statistical test of whether or not the means of several groups are equal, and therefore generalizes the t-test to more than two groups.

➤ Measures the difference between the means of three or more groups.

Chi-Square (χ2)

➤ Measures the difference between the percentages or proportions of independent variables within a large sample (not the mean values).

➤ If a smaller sample size and measuring the proportions, use **Fisher's exact test**.

Correlation coefficient (r²)

• Positive 1 = <u>strong</u> positive correlation. This indicates that as one variable increases, the other variable would also increase.

• Negative 1 = <u>strong</u> negative correlation. This indicates that as one variable increases, the other variable would decrease.

- A negative 0.5 indicates a <u>weak</u> negative correlation.
- A positive 0.5 indicates a <u>weak</u> positive correlation.
- A (0) indicates there is <u>no</u> correlation.
- If want to solve the correlation coefficient, calculate the square of (r). For example, if (r) is equal to (-0.80), -0.8 × -0.8 = .64 or 64%.

Basically: (-1)----- (-0.5) ----- (0) ----- (+0.5)---- (+1). Values always follows between -1 and +1.

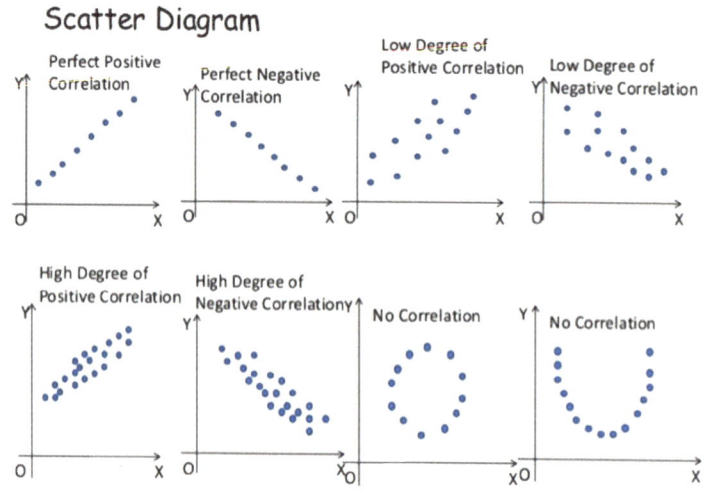

Source: www.slideshare.net

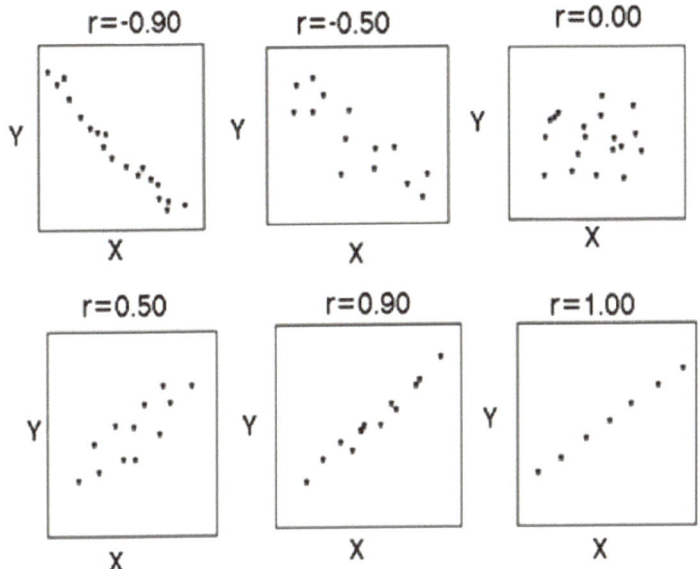

Source: www.simplypsychology.org

Correlation Coefficient
Shows Strength & Direction of Correlation

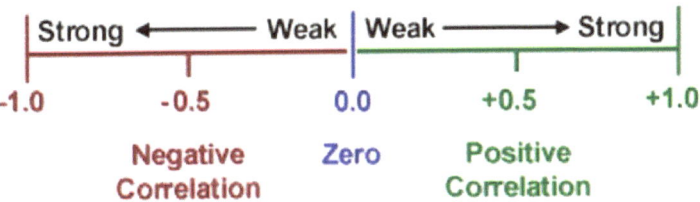

Source: psychlopedia.wikispaces.com

Preventive Medicine

Disease prevention

Prevention types: "PDR" prevention, detection, and Rx (treatment).

➤ **Primary prevention**: prevention of the disease helps decrease incidence and prevalence.

   Examples: vaccinations, exercise, dietary education, drug education, and alcohol education.

➤ **Secondary prevention**: detection of the disease.

   Example: screening for diseases.

➤ **Tertiary prevention**: reduce disability (medications).

   Examples: physical therapy, rehabilitation, and follow-up.

Most prevalent cancer types

➤ Men: prostate cancer (1st), lung cancer (2nd), and colorectal cancer (3rd).
➤ Women: breast cancer (1st), lung cancer (2nd), and colorectal cancer (3rd).

Most common cancers associated with mortality

➤ Men: lung cancer (1st), prostate cancer (2nd), and colorectal cancer (3rd).
➤ Women: lung cancer (1st), breast cancer (2nd), and colorectal cancer (3rd).

Most common gynecological cancer

➤ Endometrial cancer is the most common gynecological cancer in women aged >45.

Most common gynecological cancer associated with mortality

➤ Ovarian cancer is the most common cause of death among gynecological cancers but accounts for only about 3% of all cancers in women. Ovarian cancers are usually found in later stages of disease which leads to increase mortality.

Leading cause of mortality by age

➤ <1 year → congenital diseases.

➤ 1–44 years → unintentional injury.

➤ 45–64 years → cancers.

➤ >65 years → heart disease.

Health screening

Colonoscopy screening

➤ If no family history of colon cancer, start screening once every 10 years in patients at 50 years of age.

➤ For high-risk patients of colon cancer, start screening at 40 years of age or start screening 10 years before first-degree relative was diagnosed (whichever comes first).

➤ Screening is recommended in African Americans beginning at 45 years of age.

➤ Screen patients with Crohn's disease 8 years after initial diagnosis and then every subsequent year.

➤ If first-degree relative diagnosed with FAP, then start screening offspring with yearly colonoscopies at 12 years of age.

➤ Patients found to have adenomatous polyps on screening sigmoidoscopy, will need full colonoscopy to rule out other adenomas.

➤ Usually recommended to stop colonoscopy screening after age 75.

Flexible sigmoidoscopy

➤ If no family history of colon cancer, start screening once every 5 years in patients at 50 years of age.

➤ If high risk of colon cancer, then screening starts at age 40 or 10 years before first-degree relative was diagnosed.

➤ If sigmoidoscopy is positive, then obtain a full colonoscopy.

Digital rectal exam and guaiac tests

➤ Conduct every year after 50 years of age or at age 40 if patient is at high risk of colon cancer (controversial).

➤ **Fecal immunochemical test** (FIT) is preferred over guaiac testing.

Abdominal aortic aneurysm (AAA) screening

➤ Abdominal ultrasonography via one-time screening in men between ages 65 to 75 whom currently smoke tobacco or have a smoking history.

Pap smears

➤ Do not screen women <21 years of age (unless: HIV positive, SLE, or immunosuppressed).

➤ Guidelines state to start screening at age 21 regardless of sexual history or onset.

➤ Pap smears are recommended every 2–3 years with cytology screening only in women aged 21–29. HPV DNA testing is not recommended for this age group.

➤ Pap smears are recommended every 5 years, if combination screening with cytology plus HPV DNA testing from age 30–65 (these are the guidelines, if three prior normal Pap smears).

➤ Possible to stop screening after age 65, if the last three Pap smears were normal.

➤ Homosexual women should have same Pap screening schedule as heterosexual women.

Note:

✓ Screen according to guidelines, if diagnosed with high-grade precancerous cervical lesion, cervical cancer, DES exposure, or immunocompromised (HIV).

✓ Pap smear is a screening test for gynecological cancers.

Mammography

➤ Start screening with mammogram every 2 years from age 50 to 75.

➤ Screening before age 50 is no longer recommended unless family history of early onset.

➤ Teaching self-breast exams are no longer recommended.

➤ Clinical breast exams are no longer recommended (controversial).

➤ Mammography done on breastfeeding women are not recommended (only visualize milk on mammogram).

Note: mammography can detect lumps that cannot be felt on physical examination.

Endometrial tissue sampling

➤ Screening is not recommended unless bleeding is observed in postmenopausal women.

Chest CT-scan screening

➤ Chest x-ray is not recommended as a screening test for lung cancer.

➤ New guidelines: conduct yearly low dose chest CT-scan for 30-pack/year smokers between the ages of 55 and 80.

• Screen if patient quit <15 years ago or is a current smoker.

• If patient quit >15 years ago, then no screening is necessary.

Note: 30 packs/year means that the patient smokes 1 pack per day for 30 years <u>or</u> 2 packs per day for 15 years.

Prostate specific antigen (PSA)

➤ Not highly recommended as a screening test (nonspecific) for prostate cancer (since many things can increase PSA levels). Elevated false positives levels can lead to unnecessary biopsies.

➤ If PSA is elevated re-check in 4-6 weeks and if still elevated, consider further evaluation.

➤ Can measure PSA starting at age 40 if at high risk or at age 50 if low risk. However, screening remains controversial.

  • Need to inform patients about risks and benefits and let them decide on screening.

  • Screening may cause risk of over diagnosis and over treatment.

➤ Digital rectal exam is still used as a screening tool for prostate cancer.

➤ African American men can start screening at age 40 since they have a greater risk than other ethnicities.

Ovarian cancer screening

➤ Screening is not recommended except for high-risk patients.

➤ Screening includes CA-125 (>35 U/mL) followed by an ovarian ultrasound.

Risk factors that lead to screening recommendation include family history, BRAC-1 mutation, Lynch syndrome or HNPCC, and dermatomyositis.

BRAC1 and BRAC2 screening

➤ Should be conducted for women with family history.

➤ Increase risk of ovarian and breast cancer.

Risk factors leading to screening recommendation: first-degree relatives diagnosed at <35 years old, multiple generations in the family having the disease, or bilateral breast cancer.

Diabetic screening

➤ Start screening healthy patients at 45 years of age (then 3-5 year intervals).

➤ If fasting glucose is positive on two separate occasions, then conduct a 75g glucose test.

➤ Screen any patient with BMI >25.

➤ Screen at any age if prior diagnosis of hypertension, obesity, hyperlipidemia, or strong family history.

Lipid panel screening

➤ Screening in healthy patients is recommended in men at age ≥35 years and women at ≥45 years.

➤ Lipid panel screening is conducted every 5 years in a healthy patients and yearly for high-risk patients.

➤ If patient is at high risk (diabetes, hypertension, obesity, or family history), then screening can begin as early as age 20.

DEXA scan screening

➤ Start screening women at 65 years of age or earlier for high-risk patients.

➤ Screen patients who obtain fractures that are out of proportion to minor trauma.

➤ Patients on high dose steroids should have a baseline DEXA scan.

Hearing and vision screening

➤ Offered at age 65 or in patients with high risk of impairment.

➤ Children are also screened at various stages of development.

Glaucoma screening

➤ Screen every 3–5 years in patients with no risk factors between 40 and 60 years of age.

➤ Screen every year after age 40 if diagnosed with elevated

intraocular pressure, diabetes, African American descent, or have family history of disease.

CAGE screening

➤ A screening test used for alcohol dependency and abuse.

➤ Screen all individuals with history of alcohol abuse and depression. Ask about CAGE: cutting down on alcohol, annoyed when asked about alcohol, guilty about alcohol, and eye opener (alcohol consumption in the morning).

➤ Studies find it's more important to ask how many times in a year an individual has had >5 drinks (males) or >4 drinks (females).

➤ Always ask patient for pros and cons of drinking. If patient does not state any cons than he/she is usually not ready to quit alcohol.

Sun protection

➤ Includes protective clothing, avoiding afternoon exposure, use of sunscreen, and adequate hydration.

Vaccinations

Live attenuated

➤ MMR (measles, mumps, and rubella), polio (sabin), yellow fever, varicella, rotavirus, and influenza (nasal).

➤ In children with egg allergy there is no contraindication for using MMR (egg based), but there is a contraindication for using influenza vaccination (also egg based).

Inactivated (killed)

➤ "RIP" rabies, influenza (injected), and polio (salk vaccine).

Conjugated vaccinations

➤ Haemophilus influenzae type B (Hib), meningococcal vaccination, and pneumoniae vaccination.

Pneumococcal vaccination

➤ Administer children <2 years of age with PCV13 (given at 2 months, 4 months, 6 months, and 12 months).

  • Do not give PPSV23 to children younger than 2 years of age.

➤ Administer to all healthy adults >65 year of age and then give booster shots every 5 years. This is a two-part vaccination given 6-12 months apart from one another.

  • First 13-valent conjugated pneumococcal vaccine [PCV13] is recommended for all adults over 65 years of age followed by the 23-valent pneumococcal polysaccharide vaccine [PPSV23].

➤ Age-independent factors: should receive vaccination if diagnosed with chronic lung disease, sickle cell disease, asplenic, chronic heart disease, COPD (including asthma), diabetes mellitus, alcoholism, immunosuppressed, or live in care facilities.

➤ PPSV23 is also recommended for use in adults 19 through 64 years of age who smoke tobacco or who have asthma.

MMR vaccination

➤ MMR vaccination should not be given to individuals <6 month of age. Usually first dose is given at 1 year of age and again at 4 years of age.

➤ MMR is a live vaccination that should be considered prior to pregnancy. Patients are recommended not to get pregnant for at least one months after vaccination. However, no case reports demonstrate harm in early pregnancy.

➤ MMR vaccination is contraindicated in immunosuppressed patients. However, the exception is vaccination is not contraindicated in HIV patients.

➤ MMR vaccination is not contraindicated in children with

egg allergies. However, need to observe patient for at least 30 minutes after vaccination is given.

➤ The CDC concludes there is no evidence to support that MMR vaccination is linked to autism.

Hepatitis B vaccination

➤ Hepatitis B vaccination is indicated to every surface antibody-negative patient (negative HBsAb).

➤ Hepatitis B vaccination is a 3-dose regiment given at birth (before discharge), 2 months, and 6 months.

➤ Mother can legally refuse vaccinations to neonate. Refusal must be documented in patient chart.

➤ If patient is HBsAb negative and subjected to a contaminated syringe from a hepatitis B positive individual:

- Then give hepatitis B immune globulin plus hepatitis B vaccination.

- However, if patient has surface antibody present than no further treatment is necessary.

➤ Children born to a non-immune hepatitis B infected mother:

- Give child hepatitis B vaccination plus hepatitis immune globulin, within 12 hours of birth.

➤ Children born to an immune hepatitis B infected mother:

- Then only the hepatitis B vaccination is required for neonate.

➤ There is no hepatitis C vaccination at this time.

Risks for hepatitis B: IV drug users, homosexual males, travel to high-risk places, dialysis, and multiple sexual partners.

Note: it is more likely to contract hepatitis B, than hepatitis C or HIV from a syringe.

Hepatitis A vaccination

➤ Indications for hepatitis A vaccination:

- IV drug use, homosexual men, or chronic liver disease.

- Vaccinate if patient has had recent exposure or patient is traveling to an endemic area.
- Good hygiene and proper sanitation can help prevent spread of hepatitis A.
- Can be administered during or before pregnancy.
- All children should receive 2 doses (6 months apart) of hepatitis A vaccination, beginning at 1 year of age.
- Once an individual has had hepatitis A infection and has recovered they cannot become infected again.

Varicella vaccination

- Recommended in children at 1 year of age and again at 4 years of age (two dose regiment).
- Administer if no history of chicken pox in the past and no contraindications.
- Live vaccination that is contraindicated in pregnancy, immunosuppressed, and severe HIV infection.
- Vaccination is encouraged in patients with no previous history of chicken pox prior to getting pregnant.
- Women who get varicella vaccine may continue to breastfeed.
- Keep in mind this vaccination is a live-attenuated vaccine that is administered with 2 doses.

Shingles vaccination

- Recommended to all patients over 60 years of age.
- People who have had shingles can receive the vaccine to help prevent future occurrences.

Meningococcal vaccination

- Recommended for patient in the military, prison, living in dorms, before starting junior high, and again before starting college.
- Recommended one dose at age 11 and a booster shot at age 16.
- Vaccination can be given as early as 2 years of age in patients who are asplenic.

- MPSV4 is the only meningococcal vaccine approved for use in people over 55.
- Booster shots may be recommended in adults who remain at increased risk.

Influenza vaccination

- Everyone 6 months and older are recommended for annual flu vaccination with rare exceptions.
- IM influenza vaccination (killed vaccine) and nasal influenza vaccination (live vaccine).
- IM influenza vaccination can be given as early as 6 months of age (if no contraindications).
- If using nasal spray influenza vaccination, do not give to children younger than 2 years of age or patients >50 years of age. Not recommended in pregnant women or immunosuppressed patients.
- Routine influenza vaccination is recommended for all women who are pregnant (in any trimester) or will be pregnant during influenza season.
- Patients with severe egg allergies should not be given the influenza vaccination, especially if less than 18 years of age.
- Patients with mild egg allergies (example hives) can receive vaccination with additional safety measures and close observation.

Rabies immunoglobulin and vaccination

- If no previous history of rabies vaccination and post-exposure to rabies, will need prophylaxis with vaccination and immunoglobulin.
  - Regiment: 4 doses of rabies vaccination (days 0, 3, 7, and 14) plus 1 dose of immunoglobulin.
- If previous vaccination to rabies and post-exposure to rabies, will require booster shot with rabies vaccination alone.
  - Regiment: 2 doses of rabies vaccination only (days 0 and 3).

Note:

✓ If attacked by <u>unprovoked animal</u>: give immediate prophylaxis.

✓ If attacked by <u>provoked animal</u>: observe animal for 10 days.

Live vaccinations

➤ Are contraindicated in pregnancy, patients on chemotherapy, and immunosuppressed patients.

➤ Nasal influenza vaccine and MMR are live attenuated virus vaccines and contraindicated during pregnancy.

➤ MMR is contraindicated in immunosuppressed patients, except can be given to patients with HIV.

➤ MMR is not contraindicated in children with egg-base allergy.

Tetanus toxoid vaccination (DTaP)

➤ If received adequate tetanus vaccination within 5 years, do nothing for clean or dirty wounds.

➤ If received tetanus vaccination >5 years ago but less <10 years ago, then give a tetanus booster.

➤ If received >10 years ago, then give tetanus vaccination for both dirty and clean wounds. Add tetanus immunoglobin for dirty wounds.

➤ DTaP is recommended in children at 2, 4, 6, and 15 months; and again at age 4-6 years.

➤ Give vaccination booster every 10 years.

➤ Can be given in the second trimester of pregnancy.

➤ Can get tetanus from bites, open wounds, feces, frost bite, and burns.

Rotavirus vaccination

➤ Rotavirus is the most common cause of diarrhea in infants and children worldwide.

➤ Rotavirus is a live vaccination given at 2 months, 3 months, and 6 months of age (3 doses).

➤ Needs to be given between 2 and 8 months of age.

Palivizumab vaccination

➤ Prevention of respiratory syncytial virus (RSV) and recommended in patients younger than 2 years with bronchopulmonary dysplasia, prematurity, and hemodynamically significant heart disease.

Patient with cancer on chemotherapy

➤ Should be vaccinated with inactivated influenza and pneumococcal polysaccharide.

Gardasil vaccination

➤ Prevents cervical cancer, anal cancer, and genital warts in women.

➤ Prevents genital warts and anal cancer in men.

➤ Recommended time for first dose is age 11–12 (1st dose), two months later (2nd dose), then at six months after original dose (3rd dose). Vaccine is a three-dose regiment.

➤ Can be given between ages 11 to 26 years of age despite previous sexual activity, genital warts, previous HPV infection, and abnormal Pap smear are not contraindications.

Note:

✓ Not recommended during pregnancy, lactating women, or immunosuppressed patients.

✓ Do not need to test for HPV prior to vaccination.

Ethics

Pain medication

➤ Titration of pain medication is determined by the comfort level of the patient. Look at vital signs to confirm levels and safety.

Indirect euthanasia

➤ It is legal for terminally ill patients everywhere in the United States. Called "**double effect**," this basically constitutes giving pain control medications to relieve pain but may result in inadvertent life shortening.

➤ **Direct Euthanasia** is always the wrong answer.

Brain dead

No signs of brain function on physical exam:

➤ Reflexes include no pupillary response (fixed pupils), no corneal reflex, no response to caloric reflex test, and no spontaneous respiration.

➤ Needs to be diagnosed by two doctors.

➤ Do not need to treat patients who are brain dead.

Court-appointed legal guardian

➤ Can use when patient has either no family or no family members who are competent.

Hospital ethics committee consultation

➤ When family cannot come to an agreement on the patient's care.

Arrange a family meeting

➤ When there is a family dispute on the patients care.

Physician-patient relationship

➤ Physicians do not have an obligation to accept a patient.

➤ Patient has the right to choose a physician.

➤ Physician has the right to refer patient to another physician if he/she decides not to treat the patient any longer. However, sufficient time should be given to the patient for transfer. If patient needs care during that transition time, the original physician cannot deny treatment.

➤ Physician can terminate relationship with patient, if another physician is willing to care for patient.

➤ If a physician is on vacation, they have legal responsibility to cover their patients with another physician.

➤ Physicians should terminate the physician-patient relationship before becoming romantically involved.

➤ A patient-psychiatrist relationship is never acceptable.

➤ Report suspected sexual misconduct to the state medical board. The state medical board will investigate the matters further. Do not investigate the matters personally, as this is not your duty.

➤ Long waiting times, should be acknowledged by physician and help validate the situation.

Patient's safety

➤ Report physicians who are intoxicated or on drugs to hospital authorities or state medical board. If perpetrator is a resident-physician, then report to program director or department chair.

➤ Physicians should only conduct treatments that are beneficial for patients.

➤ Physicians can act as a moral surrogate for the benefit of a patient's health.

➤ Physicians should always obtain enough information to make a diagnosis.

➤ Always focus the patient on information useful to conduct a proper diagnosis.

Physician's safety

➤ If physician is at risk of contracting a disease from patient, then the physician needs to take extreme precautions. Patient's needs should still be addressed and patient should not be denied treatment.

➤ A physician who does not want to treat a patient with HIV with an open wound can deny treatment <u>legally</u> but it is not <u>ethical</u> to do so.

Patient records

➤ Records are the property of the patient and they have the right to see them. A written release of the records from patient is required.

➤ It is always best to go over charts together to clarify medical documents.

➤ Print out communication via emails and letters from patients/physicians and place them in patients' charts.

➤ Patient going to new physician—medical records can be shared with both patient and new physician, upon patient's request.

➤ Physicians should encourage their own family members to have their own physicians and should not treat family members.

Confidentiality

➤ Ask relatives to leave the room while breaking bad news.

➤ Do not discuss patient's information in public settings such as elevators.

➤ Confidentiality can be breached if danger to self, others, elderly abuse, or child abuse.

➤ A husband who wants to know about his wife's medical condition should ask his wife. If the husband is at risk of a medical condition, then a breach may be considered.

➤ A physician cannot obtain medical records from other doctors without direct consent.

Blood transfusions

➤ If patient refuses blood transfusions, then consider high dose IV fluids.

➤ Be aware that albumin is also considered a blood product.

➤ Pregnant women can refuse blood transfusions during pregnancy.

HIV status

➤ Persuading patients to tell their sexual partners is the first step. Some states allow doctors to tell patients' spouses (if patients refuse disclosure).

➤ All states require that you report HIV to the CDC.

➤ Physicians are allowed to give sterile needles to IV drug users.

➤ It is acceptable to ask patients in homosexual relationships if the patient is the penetrating partner or the penetrated partner (since person who is being penetrated has a higher risk of HIV secondary to tissue tearing).

➤ Physicians (surgeons) with HIV do not need to disclose to patients or co-workers their HIV status but they should take special precautions. They should tell the hospital authorities.

Research in adults

➤ Patients should always be aware if they are being studied and written consent should always be given.

➤ Prisoners being studied should have equal rights and same compensation offered as general population.

Research in children

➤ Children can refuse to participate in research studies; even in the case where parents want them to participate in the study.

➤ If a 15-year-old adolescent wants to be in a research study but parents disagree, then the child cannot participate.

➤ If both parents and children agree, they can participate.

➤ A 17-year-old adolescent who lives alone and has a child does not need parents' consent to join a research study.

Sexual misconduct

➤ Should always be reported and an official report written to hospital authorities.

Pelvic examination

➤ Male physicians: always have a female chaperon during both adolescent and adult examinations. A chaperon is also needed for sedated patients.

➤ Female physicians: always have a male chaperon during both adolescent and male examinations. A chaperon is also needed for sedated patients.

Good Samaritan law

➤ If a physician picks up a patient from an MVA and brings him/her to the ER in his/her personal car and the physical examination in the ER reveals quadriplegia, then the physician is liable for this consequence since he/she did not protect the patient's neck.

Insurance companies

➤ Require proof that hospitalization was justified and necessary.

➤ Hospitals cannot refuse patients who do not have insurance.

Gifts

➤ Physicians can accept modest gifts from patients.

➤ Extravagant gifts are never acceptable.

Homeopathic medicine

➤ For non-life-threatening conditions, patients currently using homeopathic medicine can be encouraged, if working for the patient.

➤ If homeopathic medications are not working for patient, then discontinue medications and give conventional medications.

New drug medications

➤ If physician prescribes a new drug and has noted side effects such as death, severe medical illness, or hospitalization; the physician should report the finding to the FDA.

➤ Pharmaceutical companies can compensate physicians for reimbursement of travel expenses and honoraria but they cannot control lecture content or slide show.

Doctor's personal issues

➤ Should never be part of the patient-doctor relationship, unless a patient asks a specific question and the doctor is willing to answer it.

Physician's personal ethics

➤ Physicians are not obligated to provide services (such as abortion, sterilization, or contraception), if they go against personal moral standards. However, they should refer patient to another physician and honor the patient's autonomy.

Smoking in adolescents

➤ Parents who want their children to stop smoking should quit smoking themselves.

Consent to minors

➤ Considered emancipated minors if in the military, married, living independently, or self-supported.

➤ Medical care for minors, neither the minor nor the parents can refuse treatment for life-threatening conditions, even in cases where religious beliefs and morals are involved.

➤ If critically ill newborn, parents have the right to withhold or withdraw life-sustaining treatment, if decision is in child's best interest.

➤ Minors are exempt from parental consent when dealing with

STDs, OCPs, pregnancy, and drug rehabilitation.

➤ Not exempt, if risk of harm to self or others.

➤ No need to reveal homosexuality to parents.

➤ If a pregnant teen wants to keep her baby but her mother insists on aborting the baby, the pregnant teen has the right to make her own decision.

➤ If a pregnant teen wants to abort the baby, she has the right to make the decision. The parents need not be informed but it is recommended to encourage the patient to inform her parents.

➤ Some states have notification laws for pregnant teens aborting baby.

➤ Do not need to inform parents for elective abortions in minors, unless patient does not have capacity to make her own decisions.

➤ Non-emergency in minors need consent from parents or guardian (only consent from one parent or guardian is sufficient).

➤ Treatment during emergency situations in minors does not need consent from patient or parents (for example, appendectomy). Nor can emergency treatments be denied by parents.

➤ Mothers can deny vaccinations to children since vaccinations hold little risk if not given.

➤ If a 16-year-old patient who lives by themselves refuses a blood transfusion, you should respect their decision, as they are emancipated.

➤ If a 7-year-old patient needs a blood transfusion and mother is against receiving the transfusion, a blood transfusion should be given, since this is a life-threatening situation.

➤ A 17-year-old father who requests for a bilateral vasectomy and who lives with his parents would not be granted surgery. The surgeon should give him less invasive alternatives.

➤ A 16-year-old mother who requests for a bilateral tubal ligation should not be granted the surgery. Less invasive alternatives should be given.

➤ If a 16-year-old male wants to donate his kidney to a friend with ESRD and his parents disagree, the physician cannot accept the kidney.

- If a 16-year-old male wants to donate his kidney to a friend with ESRD and his parents agree, then he can donate one kidney.

- If a child with terminal cancer wants to stop chemotherapy but the parents want to continue, then the parents' wishes should be upheld.

- Blood transfusions from siblings should be accompanied by parental consent. Unless emergency.

- Children have the right to know about their personal health care.

- If parents do not want a physician to tell their child about the child's health, the physician should respect the child's rights to know as long as the child has the capacity to understand the situation.

Child abuse

- Admit child to pediatric ward, examine completely, and consult child protective services and the psychology department.

- All children should be removed from the household.

- Most common cause of vaginal bleeding in children is the introduction of a foreign body, but also need to rule out **sarcoma botryoides**.

- If conducting a pelvic exam, sedation is needed.

Elderly abuse

- Most likely associated with physical and mental impairment in the elderly patient.

- Always separate patient from abuser (hospitalization).

- Elderly abuse needs to be considered in frail and vulnerable adults.

Drug use during pregnancy

- Report to child welfare department if urine toxicology is positive.

- If aware of mother using drugs during pregnancy, be careful with reporting because the mother might not return for future maternal visits, which is also important for both baby and mother.

Suicidal teens

➤ Need to conduct family meeting with the intention of inpatient care.

Surrogate parents

➤ Patients have unrestricted rights to donate sperm or eggs and <u>can</u> be paid for them. This is unlike for <u>organs</u>, where the donor cannot be paid.

➤ Situation: a pregnant surrogate mother signed a surrogacy contract with a couple. The couple provided the sperm and ovum. The surrogate mother wants to void the contract and she has no genetic relation to the couple.

  • Is she allowed to breach the contract? The answer is no, since the genetic parents have exclusive custody and parental rights.

➤ <u>Situation</u>: a pregnant surrogate mother signed a surrogacy contract with a couple and the couple gets divorced. The male partner provided the sperm and the female partner provided the ovum, and they decided not to continue with the surrogate pregnancy.

  • The couple has the right <u>not</u> to continue with the pregnancy.

➤ Situation: a pregnant surrogate mother signed a surrogacy contract with a couple. The couple gets divorced and the male partner gave the sperm and the surrogate mother provided the ovum. The father wants to terminate the pregnancy and the surrogate mother wants to continue.

  • The rights of the surrogate mother would be respected.

Artificial insemination

➤ Physicians cannot conduct sex selection (gender preference) except for genetic X-linked disease purposes.

Consent in adults

➤ No medical intervention should be conducted without informed consent (investigational, cosmetic, diagnostic, palliative, or therapeutic).

➤ Consent can be given verbally or signed but always better to have a signed consent form.

➤ Pelvic exams under anesthesiology need to be consented prior to giving them. Be very careful with this one.

➤ Patients can withdraw consent at any time.

➤ Patient needs to be mentally competent and completely informed about risks, benefits, and alternative treatments.

➤ Patient needs to understand the language.

➤ Psychiatric patients who are competent can consent to procedures as long as they understand the risks and benefits. If patients do not understand the procedure then they can ask a relative or obtain a court order.

➤ Suicidal patients are automatically marked as <u>not</u> having decision-making capacity.

➤ If patient, has decision-making capacity for a <u>life-threatening</u> procedure in the morning and accepts the procedure but in the afternoon loses their decision-making capacity and denies the procedure, respect the morning decision and perform the procedure.

➤ If a diabetic patient who needs an amputation from gangrene reports to hospital saying she is fine and has no medical problems, then consent from family member for amputation is needed.

➤ Down's syndrome patient living on their own who understands the procedure can make their own decisions.

➤ If a mentally retarded woman wants to keep her baby but her husband and mother want an abortion, respect the mother's wishes if the patient is competent.

Organ donors

➤ Should not receive large sums of money for donations but are allowed to receive money for medical expenses.

> HIV patients cannot donate organs.

> Driver's licenses of organ donors must be confirmed by family members.

> Organs from an organ donor with an expired card cannot be accepted unless approved by family.

Proxy advance directive

> Decision makers in order of priority: spouse → adult child → parent → sibling → relative or concerned friend. If none are available then a public official may serve as a decision maker.

> The Health Care Proxy is the strongest advance directive.

Negligence

> To prove the care provided by the doctor was below the appropriate standard of care and this caused the patient harm.

Gay or lesbian parents

> Children show no differences in psychosocial development.

Medical students

> Should not introduce themselves, as "doctors," and patient should be aware of medical procedures conducted by medical students. Patients have the right to refuse procedures from students or from any one for that matter.

> Medical students and residents can refuse instructions by attending physician, if they feel the instructions are inappropriate or not indicated. Always communicate with attending physician or supervisor.

> Report all mistakes to attending physicians and patients.

Disclosure

> Patients have the right not to be informed about their diagnosis.

> Always disclose errors to the patients; most effectively done by personal contact.

- Errors do not necessarily constitute improper behavior, but negligent, unethical behavior, or failure to disclose errors to patients may.

- Need to disclose, if a patient threatens to kill someone. Need to report to local police department.

- If a patient has epilepsy and is applying for a bus driving job, the physician should disclose the condition to the employer.

- If a patient has an autosomal dominant disease, the physician can disclose disease to significant other if the couple is interested in having children.

- Patients should always be well informed about all aspects of their health.

Persistent vegetative state

- Physician can decide in most states to discontinue nutrition and hydration for these patients.

Hospice care

- Is an option for terminal conditions, with an estimated prognosis of less than 6 months.

- Goals are to maximize comfort and lifestyle goals.

- Hospice does not mean do not treat, nor does it mean that patients cannot be on full code status.

Against medical advice (AMA)

- Patients have the right to leave AMA except if they propose harm to self or others.

- If patient is intoxicated or risks harm to self or others, they can be placed under physical restraint.

Do not resuscitate/Do no intubate (DNR/DNI)

- If patient is competent, can cancel DNR/DNI at any time.

- Orders allow competent individuals to express their preferences for future care.

- If patient's DNR/DNI is not available in an emergency situation, then treatment would outweigh spending valuable time looking through charts and family contacts for information.

➤ DNR/DNI orders should always be written in patients' charts.

➤ If <u>only</u> a DNI order is given, then you still need to resuscitate patient if needed.

➤ Patients or health care proxy have the right to remove all fluids and nutrition.

➤ DNR/DNI does not equal do not treat.

Best of luck on your EXAM!!!

Gregory Fernandez M.D.

Index

A

abdominal aortic aneurysm screening 33
accuracy 21
against medical advice (AMA) 56
alternative (H1) 24
analysis of variance (ANOVA) 27
arrange a family meeting 45
artificial insemination 53
attributable risk 10, 19

B

bell-shaped curve 14
Berkson's bias 6, 8
bias types 6
bimodal 24
biostatistics 9
blind studies 5
blood transfusions 48, 52
BRAC1 and BRAC2 screening 35
brain dead 45

C

CAGE screening 37
case-control study 2, 17
case report 5
chest CT-scan screening 34
child abuse 52
chi-square (χ2) 27
clinical trial 3
cohort study 1, 2, 17, 18, 19
colonoscopy screening 32
common types of bias 6
confidentiality 47
confounding bias 9
conjugated vaccinations 38
consent in adults 54
consent to minors 50
correlation coefficient (r^2) 27
court-appointed legal guardian 45
crossover studies 4
cross-sectional study 4

D

DEXA scan screening 36
diabetic screening 36
digital rectal exam and guaiac tests 33
direct euthanasia 45
disclosure 55
disease prevention 31
doctor's personal issues 50
do not resuscitate/Do no intubate (DNR/DNI) 56
double-blind study 5
double effect 45
drug use during pregnancy 52

E

euthanasia 45
effect modification 6
elderly abuse 52
endometrial tissue sampling 34

F

fecal immunochemical test 33
Fisher's exact test 27
flexible sigmoidoscopy 33

G

Gardasil vaccination 43
gay or lesbian parents 55
gifts 49
glaucoma screening 36
Good Samaritan law 49

H

Hawthorne 6, 8
health screening 32
hearing and vision screening 36
hepatitis B and A vaccination 39
HIV status 48
homeopathic medicine 49
hospice care 56
hospital ethics committee 45

Index, continued

I

inactivated vaccinations 37
incidence 20
indirect euthanasia 45
influenza vaccination 41
insurance companies 49
intention-to-treat 9

L

late-look bias 8
latent period 5, 6
leading cause of mortality by age
32
lead-time bias 8
lipid panel screening 36
live attenuated 37
live vaccinations 42
longitudinal study 3

M

mammography 34
mean 21, 23, 24
measuring bias 6
median 21, 22
medical students 55
meningococcal vaccination 40
meta-analysis 5
MMR vaccination 38, 39
mode 21, 22
most common cancers associated
with mortality 31
most common gynecological cancer
31, 32
most common gynecological cancer
associated with mortality 32
most prevalent cancer types 31

N

negative predictive value 16
negative skew 24
negligence 55
new drug medications 50

normal bell shape 22
null hypothesis 24
number needed to harm 19
number needed to treat 9
numbers needed to harm 10

O

observational bias 7
odds ratio 16
organ donors 54
ovarian cancer screening 35

P

pain medication 45
paired t-test 27
palivizumab vaccination 43
pap smears 33
patient records 47
patient's safety 46
patient with cancer on chemotherapy 43
pelvic examination 49
persistent vegetative state 56
physician-patient relationship 46
physician's personal ethics 50
physician's safety 47
pneumococcal vaccination 38
positive predictive value 15
positive skew 23
power (1-β) 25
precision 21
prevalence 16, 19, 21
primary prevention 20, 31
procedure bias 5
prospective cohort study 1, 3
prostate specific antigen 35
proxy advance directive 55
Pygmalion 6, 8

R

rabies immunoglobulin and vaccination 41
randomization 6

Epidemiology In Your Pocket

Index, continued

range 21, 22
recall bias 7
relative risk 1, 17, 18
reporting bias 7
research in adults 48
research in children 48
retrospective cohort study 1
rotavirus vaccination 42

S

sampling bias 7
secondary prevention 31
selection bias 7, 8
sensitivity 10, 11
sexual misconduct 49
shingles vaccination 40
single-blind study 5
smoking in adolescents 50
specificity 12
statistical distribution 21
stratified analysis 9
study designs 1
suicidal teens 53
sun protection 37
surrogate parents 53

T

tertiary prevention 31
tetanus 42
T-test (student's t-test) 27
type 1 error (α) 24
type II error (β) 25

V

vaccinations 37
validity 5, 12, 21
Varicella vaccination 40

Z

Z-score 22, 26

www.ingramcontent.com/pod-product-compliance
Lightning Source LLC
Chambersburg PA
CBHW040843180526
45159CB00001B/300